MARGARET TEBO

Eating Vs Drinking Your Fruits

A Comparative Guide to Optimal Fruit Consumption to Enhance Health and Wellness

This book was professionally typeset on Reedsy.
Find out more at reedsy.com

Contents

Introduction

Convenience frequently trumps nutrition in today's fast-paced world. This is why it is more common to see many people grab a bottle or glass of fruit juice than a piece of whole fruit. The argument between eating fruits whole and drinking fruit-based beverages has become more relevant than ever in our present health-conscious society. Although fruit juices are advertised as a healthy fruit consumption option compared to whole fruits, things are truly more complex than meets the eye. While whole fruits might seem interchangeable with fruit juices, they differ vastly in their nutritional profiles and the health benefits they bestow.

Whole fruits are a powerhouse of nutrients, packed with several minerals and vitamins such as vitamins C and A, potassium, and folate. They are generally cholesterol-free and low in calories, fat, and sodium. In addition, whole fruits contain great amounts of dietary fiber, which is essential for weight loss, weight management, blood sugar control, digestion, and gut health. On the other hand, fruit-based beverages tend to contain little or no fiber, as most of the fiber is removed during the juice-making process. Also, taking out fiber allows for the concentration of natural sugars during the juice-making process resulting in different metabolic responses in the body such as a rapid increase in blood sugar, and weight gain amongst others.

The principal goal of this book is to bring to light the differences in nutrient content and health outcomes between whole fruit and fruit juice consumption. By providing you with a comprehensive comparison between the two, this book will equip you with the right knowledge to enable you to make informed diet decisions. This book will also give you everyday tips to aid you in incorporating more whole fruits into your diet and give you great recommendations for fruit juice consumption.

1

Nutritional Profile of Fruits

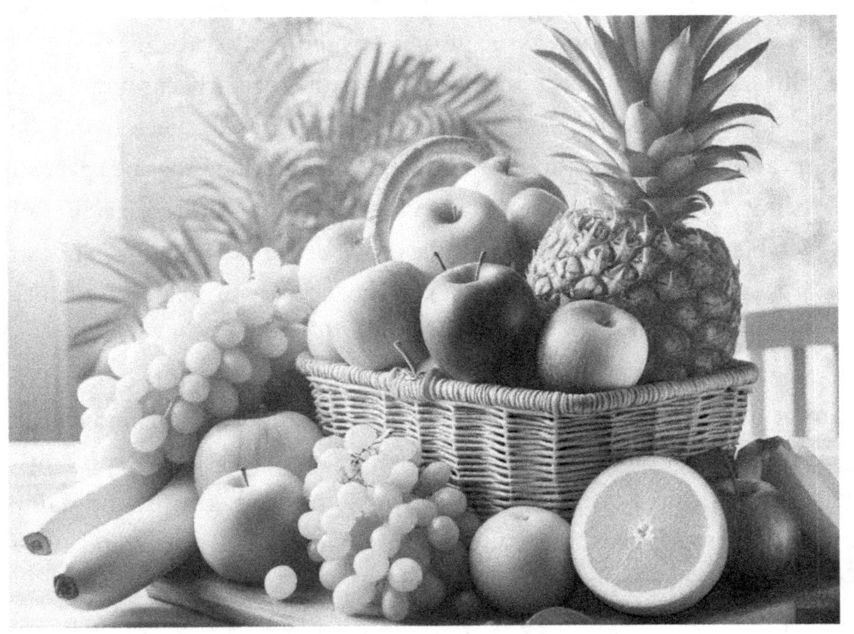

A basket of fruits on a table

Why Fruits?

Fruits have always been a part of the human diet from time immemorial. Before the dawn of agriculture and plant domestication, hunter-gatherers would hunt wild fruits alongside meat, fish, vegetables, nuts, and seeds. There still exist some Indigenous tribes who feed heavily on fruits like the Amazon people who mainly eat manioc, fish from the local rivers, and an exotic variety of tropical fruits.

Today people eat fruits for various reasons, with health being the foremost. The regular consumption of fruits and vegetables has been a steady recommendation from dietitians and other healthcare professionals for years and years now. With research studies continually demonstrating a strong association between fruit consumption and health status, the emphasis on consuming fruits regularly has intensified. For instance, one large study conducted by researchers from the Harvard T. H. Chan School of Public Health revealed that people can live longer if they consume two servings of fruit and three servings of vegetables daily. Several other studies have proven that people who eat more fruits and vegetables have a significantly lower risk of mortality from all causes, especially cardiovascular disease.

Fruits make up one of the five food groups that are an integral part of any healthy diet plan. The graphic nutrition guide established by the USDA (United States Department of Agriculture), MyPlate, portrays five food groups: fruits, vegetables, protein foods, grains, and dairy. According to MyPlate, the Fruit Group consists of every fruit and 100% fruit juice. The picture below depicts a typical MyPlate model.

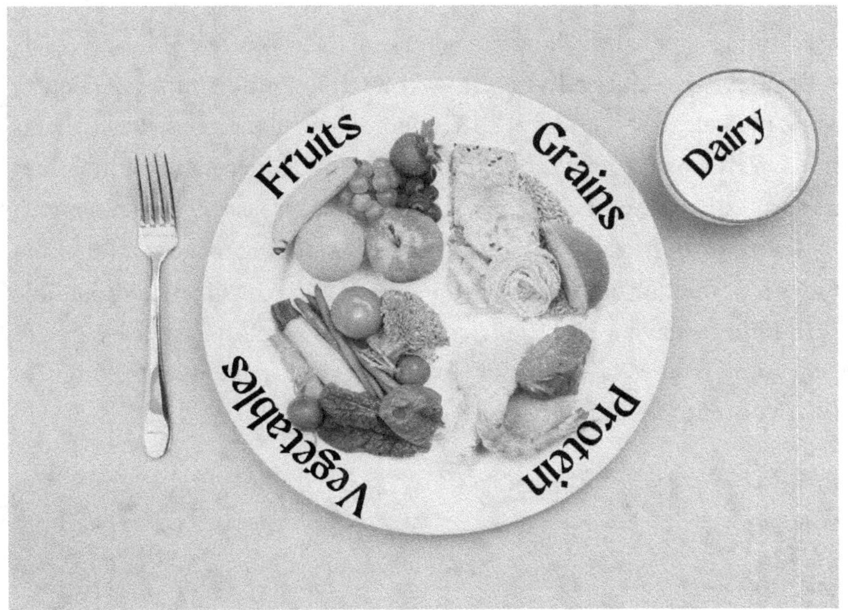

MyPlate food model

Nutrition Profile of Fruits

The primary content of fruits is water, with most fruits containing at least 81% water. Fruits are also a powerhouse of minerals and vitamins, predominantly vitamins C and A, potassium, and folate. Minerals and vitamins are micronutrients that our bodies need for proper functioning. They are called micronutrients because they are not required in large quantities in the body. However, their deficiency can result in mild-to-severe diseases or malfunctioning of the different body cells, tissues, or organs. A deficiency in vitamin C for example results in a disease or condition called scurvy which leads to poor healing of wounds or cuts. This is because vitamin C is essential for the proper growth and repair of all body tissues. It is also needed to produce collagen, the protein used to make cartilage, ligaments, tendons, the skin, and blood vessels.

Besides minerals and vitamins, fruits are a good source of dietary fiber, typically between 3.9 – 6.1%. Fiber is a type of carbohydrate that is not digested by the enzymes of our human intestine. As a result, it does not add calories to our diet. This is one of the reasons why fiber-rich foods are revolutionary in weight loss and weight management therapy. Fiber is abundant in the backs or peels of fruits, thus fruits with edible skin tend to have a high fiber content. This includes berries, guava, pears, and prunes. The chart below shows the fruits with the highest fiber content, measured per one-cup serving.

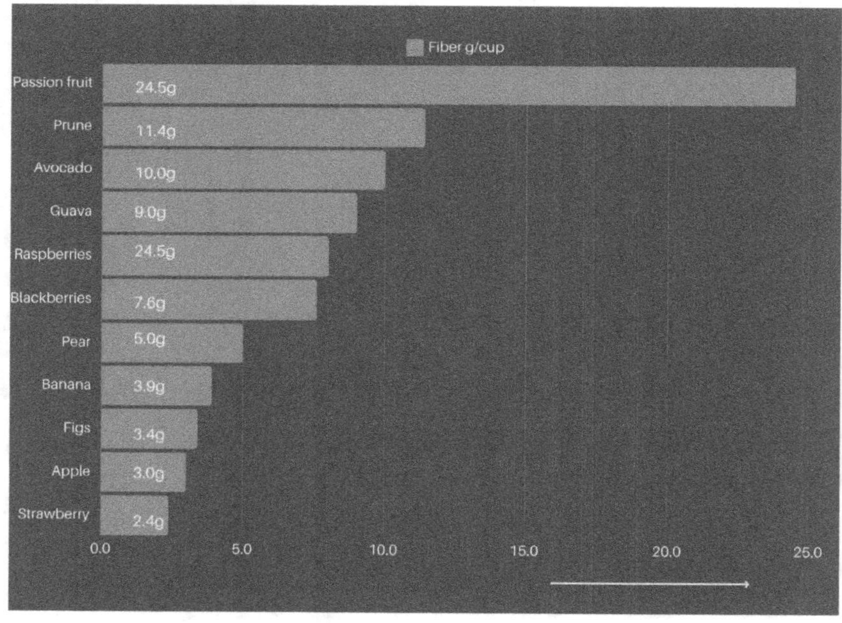

Bar chart showing the fiber content of different fruits

In addition to minerals, vitamins, and fiber, fruits are an excellent source of naturally occurring chemical compounds called phytonutrients (phytochemicals) such as polyphenols, carotenoids, phytosterols, and saponins. These compounds have biological activities that are beneficial to the body such as antioxidant, anti-inflammatory, anti-analgesic, anti-viral, anti-microbial, and cancer-protective activities. Blackberries contain the highest quantity of polyphenols with 80 – 270 milligrams of polyphenols in a 100-gram serving.

Fruits are low in calories, carbohydrates (4.3 – 10 %), protein (0.75 – 3.7%) and contain negligible amounts of lipids (0.4 – 0.55%).

2

Health Benefits of Fruits

The presence of minerals, vitamins, fiber, and phytonutrients in fruits makes them a superfood group. The following are some of the established health benefits of fruits.

Help prevent chronic diseases

The polyphenols in fruits are potent antioxidants, which protect the body's cells from damage. Antioxidants are compounds that scout and capture or neutralize free radicals (very unstable and reactive atoms), capable of harming the DNA, cell membranes, and other cell parts. Such damages can cause cell death and other modifications in regular metabolism that can bring about disease in the body. Thus, by capturing these free radicals, antioxidants can prevent excessive cellular reactions that cause damage to the cells and put the body in a state of oxidative stress. Oxidative stress is the root cause of many chronic diseases like diabetes, cancer, cardiovascular disease, and arthritis. It is also implicated in the development of neurodegenerative diseases like Alzheimer's, Huntington's, and Parkinson's disease.

Ease/prevent constipation

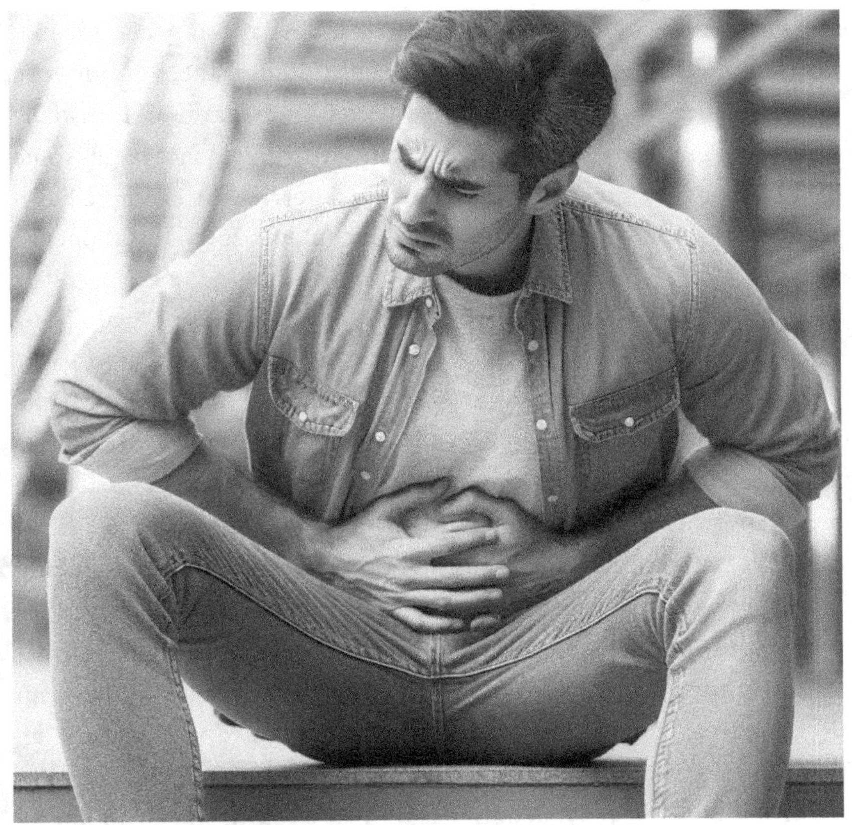

Man holding his stomach in pain

The high fiber content of fruits makes them good natural laxatives. Dietary fiber exists in two categories: soluble and insoluble fiber. Soluble fiber dissolves in water when consumed whereas insoluble fiber does not. Instead, insoluble fiber pulls water from the intestines, increasing the volume and bulk of feces. This makes feces soft and easy to pass out, increasing bowel movements and hence decreasing the probability of constipation. Constipation can cause abdominal pain, bloating, and sluggish feelings. Chronic constipation can result in more serious complications like hemorrhoids (piles), rectal prolapse, anal fissures, and bowel incontinence (leakage of liquid stools). Adults are therefore encouraged to consume between 22 – 34 grams of fiber daily depending on their age and sex, and fruits are a great place to get some of this fiber recommended. A cup of blackberries for example has 8 grams of fiber, and a cup of passion fruit contains 25 grams of fiber.

Help reduce blood cholesterol

Fruits have zero cholesterol and saturated fat, so consuming fruits regularly does not increase cholesterol levels. In addition, fiber binds to cholesterol molecules in the small intestine and prevents them from being absorbed into the bloodstream. The fiber-bound cholesterol complex is then excreted from the body in feces, directly reducing blood cholesterol levels. Apples, pears, and citrus fruits like oranges and lemons all contain pectin (a type of soluble fiber) making them great for lowering blood cholesterol levels. Fiber binding to cholesterol can decrease total blood cholesterol by 5 – 16% without affecting the HDL (high-density lipoprotein) cholesterol, which is the good cholesterol.

Furthermore, the polyphenols in fruits play a role in blood cholesterol control. Anthocyanins in raspberries and lycopene in watermelon can reduce LDL (low-density lipoprotein) cholesterol which is the bad cholesterol responsible for the development of cardiovascular disease. High blood cholesterol also called hyperlipidemia, is a major risk factor for the onset of atherosclerosis, chronic kidney disease, heart attack, and stroke which all account for millions of deaths yearly in the United States and globally.

Aid weight loss/management

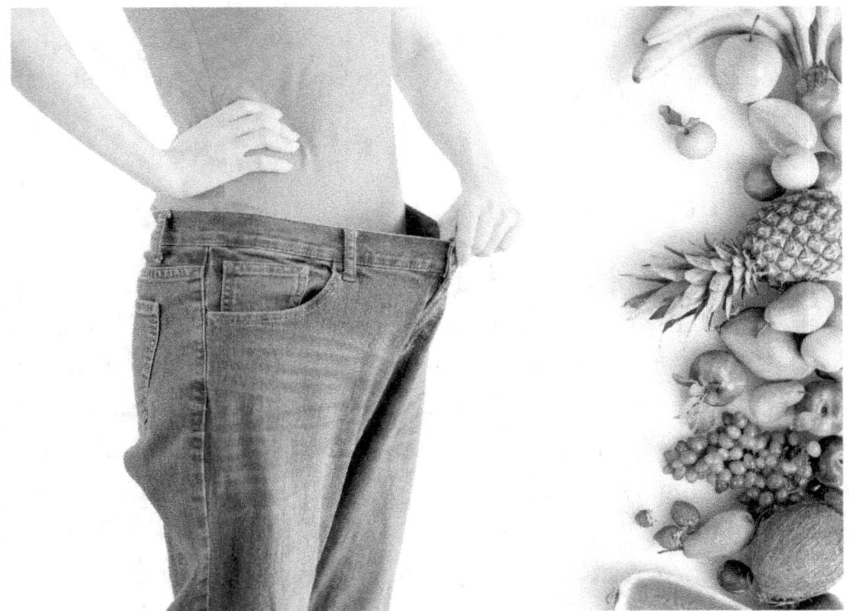

A woman in big jean pants with fruits at the side

Fruits are low in calories and fat, which makes them ideal for any weight management or weight loss program. For example, watermelons contain only 30 calories per 100g serving, peaches contain 42 calories per 100g serving and apples contain 52 calories per 100g serving. Moreover, fruits are a good source of fiber that influences weight loss/maintenance in a couple of ways. As mentioned earlier, fiber is a type of carbohydrate which is not digested because our intestine lacks the enzymes to break it down. Hence, fiber does not supply calories or energy to the body, making fruits a great addition to any weight loss or maintenance diet plan. Besides soluble fiber in fruits dissolves in water forming a thick viscous gel that slows down the exit of food from the stomach. By slowing down the exit of food from the stomach, fiber can keep you feeling full for a longer period, which helps you decrease calorie intake and overeating. This sustained satiety effect is another reason fiber-rich foods are incorporated into weight loss or management diet plans.

Help hydrate the body

Most fruits contain a significant amount of water hence, consuming them is a healthy way of taking in water and keeping oneself hydrated. Cantaloupe, honeydew, and watermelons all contain at least 90% water, while oranges, pineapples, peaches, and grapes all contain at least 85% water. Therefore, eating fruits can help you make up your daily water intake. Staying hydrated is important because water is vital for the proper functioning of each cell, tissue, and organ of the body. Water is needed to help regulate body temperature, lubricate joints, remove body waste, transport nutrients and oxygen around the body, and protect vital organs. Besides, water is the major constituent of blood, so blood decreases in volume and thickens if a person is dehydrated. This can cause a drop in blood pressure and consequently dizziness and fainting.

Boost gut health

Fiber in fruits has beneficial effects on gut health and overall immunity. Since fiber reaches the large intestines intact, it becomes food for the good bacteria that naturally live there. Bacteroides and Firmicutes are the main groups of good bacteria that feed on undigested food remains. These bacteria feed on the fiber, multiply, and phase off the bad disease-causing bacteria. When they digest fiber, they produce by-products like short-chain fatty acids and lactate that reduce the pH of the intestines (making the intestine pH more acidic). This inhibits the growth of disease-causing bacteria which typically thrive better in a neutral pH environment. Furthermore, other by-products of fiber digestion like ammonia gas and indoles are toxic to pathogenic bacteria, limiting their growth and proliferation.

The proportion of healthy bacteria to disease-causing bacteria is crucial to determining host immunity. Ideally, a healthy gut typically has a ratio of 80 – 85% good bacteria to 15 – 20% bad bacteria. Any disruption of this balance in favor of the bad bacteria results in digestive disorders like constipation, diarrhea, leaky gut, or IBS (irritable bowel syndrome). This is the reason why the consumption of probiotic foods has increased significantly nowadays because they contain live microorganisms whose target is to improve the good bacteria population. Thus, consuming fruits is one affordable way of getting great probiotic effects thanks to their rich fiber content. A leaky gut can cause poor absorption of nutrients leading to deficiencies that can affect health negatively in the long run.

Can help prevent certain cancers

Insoluble fiber draws water from the intestines and increases bowel movements. By increasing bowel movements, fiber reduces the time cancer-causing compounds (carcinogens) spend in contact with the large intestines. This helps to prevent or reduce the risk of developing colorectal cancer. Besides, by drawing water from the intestines, insoluble fiber dilutes these carcinogens, reducing their concentrations and potential to cause damage or develop cancer in the large intestine. Additionally, some polyphenols in fruits have cancer-protective abilities which they exhibit in a couple of ways. They can inhibit tumor cell growth by causing the cells to age. They also can stop cancer cell division and mutation by disrupting communication between the cells. Moreover, they kill the cells by inducing automatic cell death (autophagy). Ellagic acid and resveratrol naturally found in berries, grapes, and wines have been demonstrated to protect from certain cancers like colon, breast, skin, liver, pancreas, and thyroid cancers.

Reduce blood pressure

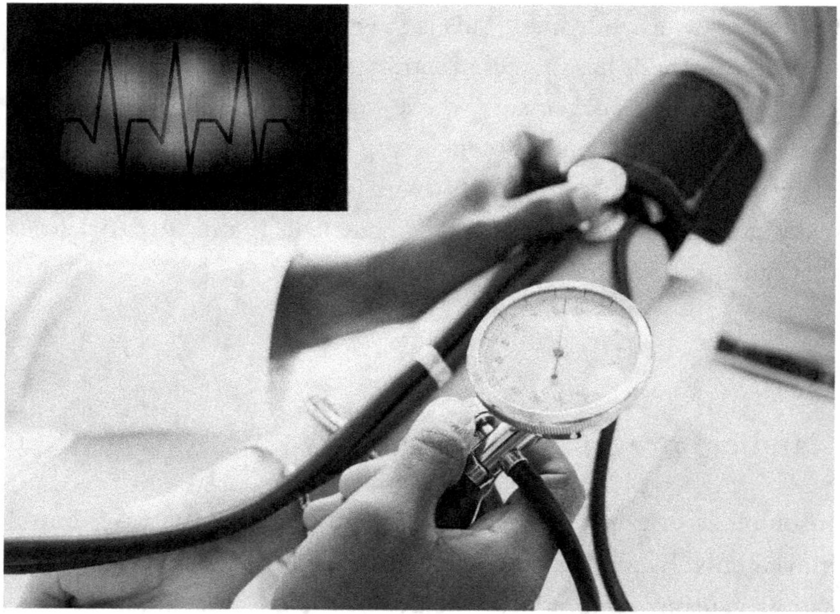

A doctor taking the blood pressure of a patient

Many fruits are a good source of potassium, which helps to reduce blood pressure by countering the effects of sodium. One medium-sized banana contains about 450 mg of potassium, which is approximately 9%

of the recommended daily intake value for potassium. Other potassium-rich fruits include prunes (732 mg), avocados (485 mg), kiwi fruit (312 mg), cantaloupe (267 mg), apricots (259 mg), and pomegranates (236 mg), all potassium levels measured per 100g serving of the fruits. High blood pressure or hypertension is a major risk factor for heart attack, stroke, kidney failure, and eye problems. Research studies have shown a reduced risk of developing high blood pressure for people who ate more whole fruits than those who did not.

Boost immunity

Fruits are an excellent source of vitamin C, which is best known for its ability to strengthen the immune system and reduce our susceptibility to infections. Vitamin C is an antioxidant, thus it enhances the skin's ability to protect the body from environmental oxidative stress. Likewise, vitamin C is used by the body to produce collagen, which gives the skin its elasticity, toughness, and bounce. This helps in the rapid healing of wounds and cuts. Similarly, vitamin C is used to produce white blood cells which are an integral part of the body's immune system. Vitamin C aids immune cells to reach the area of bacterial infection quicker and further helps them eliminate the microbes causing the infections. Besides, vitamin C is needed for the growth and repair of all the cells and tissues of the body. A deficiency in vitamin C increases host susceptibility to infection and slows down the healing of wounds.

3

Eating Vs Drinking Fruits

After expounding on the numerous health benefits of consuming fruits, it now becomes expedient to know how best to consume them to maximize all these health benefits. Some people argue that eating fruits whole is best, while others believe that drinking your fruits is best. In this chapter, we will explore the benefits and drawbacks of each method of fruit consumption.

Eating Fruits Whole

Eating fruits whole entails consuming them intact. This has been the traditional way of consuming fruits since time immemorial. People would grab their fruits and eat them as is. Here are some benefits and drawbacks of eating fruits whole.

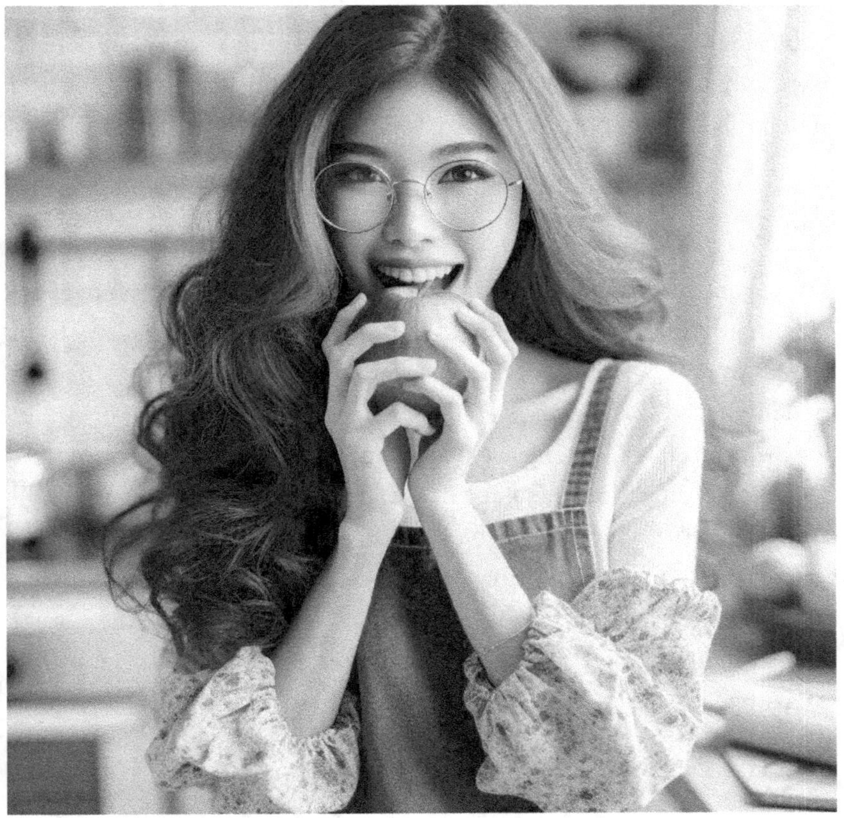

A lady biting on an apple

Benefits

More fiber

The fiber in fruits is more abundant in the peels than in the juice. A medium whole apple for example contains 4.4 grams of fiber, whereas the apple without peels contains 2.1 grams. In addition, the pulp or pomace of fruits also has plenty of fiber. Hence eating these fruits whole increases a person's fiber consumption making them benefit more from all the numerous health benefits of fiber already discussed in the previous chapter.

Calorie intake control

Eating your fruits whole tends to regulate calorie intake. This is because chewing or mastication suppresses hunger and promotes satiety in several ways. Chewing activates the centers of the brain that suppress food intake thus promoting satiety. Also, chewing your food more times per bite can boost the release of gut hormones like cholecystokinin, peptide YY, glucagon-like peptides, and insulin. These hormones all control appetite which helps you reduce calorie intake. This is why it is generally recommended to chew your food properly before swallowing. So, chewing fruits makes you consume less. Additionally, the higher fiber content of whole fruits also contributes to keeping you feeling full for a longer time as soluble fiber dissolves in water and slows down the exit of food from the stomach.

Blood sugar control

Since fruits are rich in fiber that is not broken down or digested, they are good for blood sugar control as they do not spike up sugar levels in the blood. Besides, soluble fiber dissolves in water when consumed and slows down the exit of food from the stomach, slowing down the digestion process as well. Slower digestion means slower absorption of glucose which does not spike blood glucose levels. Such action is beneficial for diabetics, the reason they are usually encouraged to eat a fiber-rich diet. Apples, bananas, grapes, berries, and apricots are some examples of fruits with a good amount of soluble fiber. A small-sized orange contains 2.9 grams of fiber, of which approximately 1.8 grams is soluble fiber, and 1.1 grams is insoluble fiber. Also, half of a small-sized fresh mango contains 2.9 grams of fiber of which 1.7 grams is soluble fiber and 1.2 grams is insoluble fiber.

Reduced nutrient losses

Eating fruits whole provides the entirety of the nutrients present without fear of losses that come with processing as is the case with commercially processed fruit drinks. Minerals, vitamins, and phytonutrients packed in the edible peels are not lost when fruits are eaten whole.

Drawback

Taste

Some fruits do not taste good when eaten alone because they are either very sour or too bland. Citrus fruits like lemons, limes, grapefruits, and pineapples have a high citric acid content, giving them a sour or sharp taste. However, these may taste better if combined with other fruits in a smoothie or homemade or processed fruit juice.

Drinking Fruit Juices

When someone says they are having fruit juice, there is an instant tendency to conclude that the person is having a fruit-filled nutritious beverage, but that is not always the case. The name "Fruit juice" is an umbrella under which different categories of fruit-based beverages sit. Based on their fruit content, fruit juices can be broadly classified into four categories: 100% fruit juice, concentrated juice, fruit nectar, and fruit drink.

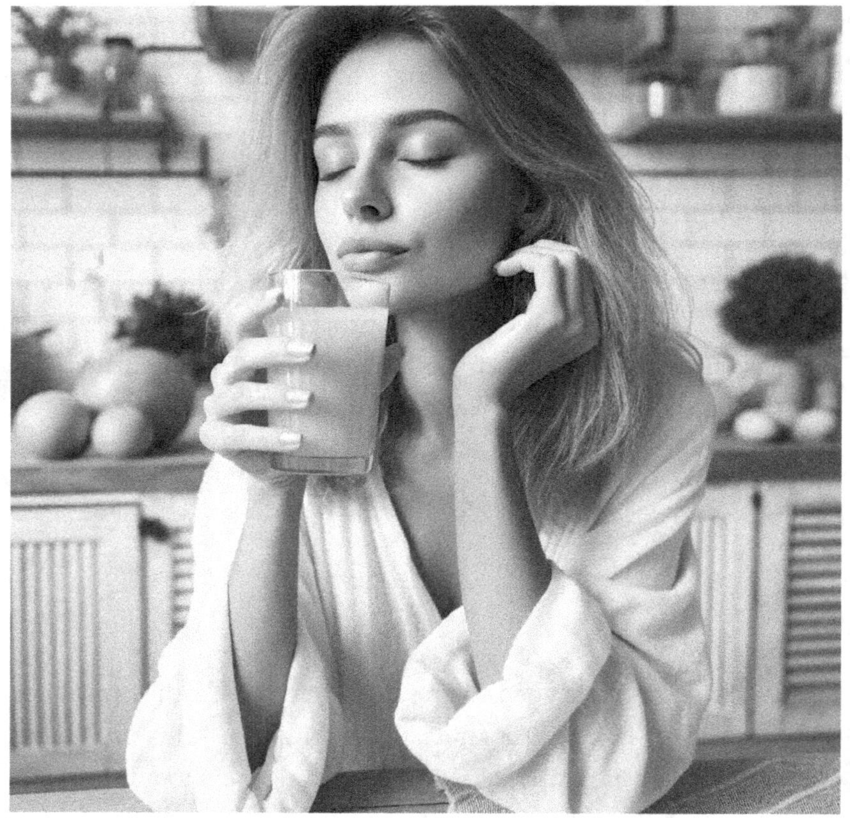

A woman drinking a glass of orange juice

A 100% fruit juice, also called crude juice, is a juice made entirely from fruits, with no added sugar. Freshly squeezed orange juice is an example of a true 100% fruit juice. Concentrated juice is crude juice whose water content has been removed. As such, fruit concentrates are very thick and high in natural sugar content. Although fruit concentrates are sometimes sold in stores, juices are mostly concentrated for easy storage and transport to production facilities. Once there, they are reconstituted to about the same solids as the original juices, packaged, and sold as 100% fruit juice from concentrates.

Fruit nectars are fruit juices diluted to contain between 25 – 50% crude juice by weight. Juice drinks including juice cocktails and juice punches, are fruit juices that contain as little as 10% or less crude juice by weight. The juice is greatly diluted and other ingredients like sugar and coloring are added to make up the fruit's taste and appearance. Unfortunately, a lot of what people consume as fruit juices are juice drinks with very little crude juice content. The picture below shows a collage of the nutrition labels of different fruit juices in grocery stores.

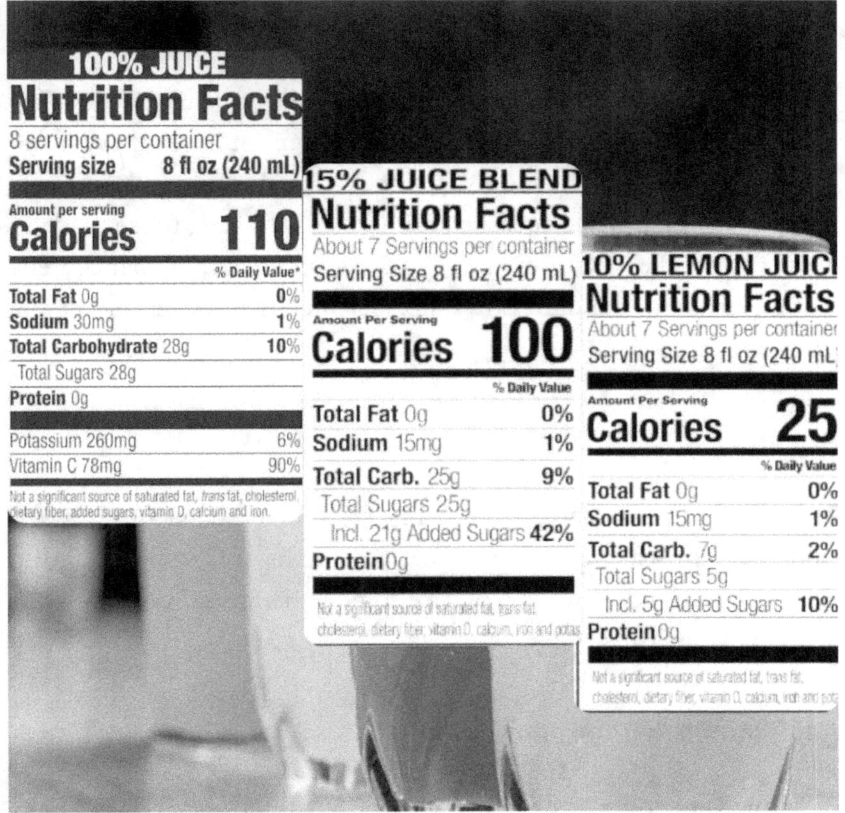

Crude juice content of different fruit juices

Processing of Fruit Juices

Though there are a plethora of fruit juices out there with several production lines, the core production steps are about the same. In the traditional production, the fruits are first sorted, washed, peeled, and crushed. Next, the juice is extracted, and it undergoes pulping and filtration to remove all suspended fruit solids, leaving a clearer juice. The filtered juice is pasteurized, or heat sterilized, cooled, and finally packaged appropriately for distribution. Depending on the type of juice being made, other ingredients such as water, sugar, sweeteners, additives, coloring agents, and preservatives, are added before pasteurizing the juice. Worth noting is that all fruit juices be they 100% fruit juice or juice drinks, have one thing in common: the removal of peels at the start of the process and the removal of fruit pulp/pomace towards the end. Therefore, all fruit juices, including those made at home with the help of juicers, have a significantly reduced fiber content, and this is the paramount difference between fruit juices and whole fruits.

Benefits

Since juices are extracted from fruits, fruit juices (particularly 100% fruit juices) provide several of the health benefits of fruit consumption already described above. Below are some benefits and downsides of drinking your fruits.

Rapid nutrient absorption

Drinking your fruits favors rapid absorption of nutrients because fiber and other components in whole fruits that slow down digestion are significantly reduced in fruit juices. This may be ideal for people recovering from certain sicknesses or surgeries, who are not yet able to chew well, yet their bodies need quick absorption of nutrients.

Quick release of sugars

The rapid absorption that comes with drinking fruits facilitates the speedy release of sugars into the bloodstream which can be advantageous in periods of low blood sugar or hypoglycemia. Drinking fruit juice can thus quickly help people (including diabetics) stabilize their blood sugar in moments of exhaustion due to physical activity or stress. Research studies show that people with type 1 diabetes mellitus drank fruit juice over 70% of the time they had episodes of hypoglycemia.

Great cocktail options

By consuming your fruits as drinks, it is possible to make a variety of combos or cocktails. Fruits are rich in diversity, so there exist endless possibilities of combinations resulting in great taste and flavors. Sweet fruits can be combined with bland fruits to give a pleasant-tasting combo. For example, sweet fruits like red grapes and mangoes can be combined with bland fruits like dragon fruit to produce a great-tasting juice. Cocktailing fruits also eases fruit consumption for sensitive people. Acidic fruits can be combined with neutral fruits to give a more soothing taste which people with teeth sensitivity can better handle. A pineapple watermelon juice for instance, will be soothing for someone with teeth sensitivity to pineapples or acidic fruits in general. Moreover, since people are encouraged to consume a variety of fruits because no one fruit has it all, cocktailing fruits makes it easy to consume a variety of fruits in one serving.

Drawbacks

Reduced fiber intake

The paramount downside of consuming fruit juices, whether home-made or commercially prepared, is reduced fiber content. During production, a substantial quantity of fiber is removed at the early step of fruit peeling. A medium-sized unpeeled apple has nearly two times more fiber than a peeled apple. Plus, the fruit pulp which also contains plenty of fiber is removed during the filtration process to make juices that are clear, and which have little or no sediments while they sit on the shelf. While it may be an esthetic quality to have clear juices, important nutrients like fiber in the peels and fruit pulp are compromised. This reduced fiber content in fruit juices robs fruit juice consumers of the optimal health benefits of fiber already mentioned in chapter one of this book. According to the USDA, 95% of people in America do not eat enough fiber, 50% consume only half of their recommended fiber and only 5% meet their recommended fiber needs.

Reduced intake of other nutrients

Besides fiber, the peels and pulp of fruits contain other important minerals, vitamins, and phytochemicals, that are also removed during the processing of fruit juices. Carotenoids, for example, are the main phytochemicals in the peels of apples, as they are responsible for the color of the fruit. Carotenoids are good antioxidants and anti-inflammatory agents that help boost our immune system, reduce swelling, and support healthy eyes, skin, and heart. Hence, throwing away apple peels greatly reduces the quantity of carotenoids consumed and consequently the antioxidant potential of the apple. Besides, a whole apple also contains about 332% more vitamin K, 40% more vitamin A, and 19% more potassium than a peeled apple. Resveratrol in red grapes which helps to stop or slow down the growth rate of tumor cells, is abundant in peels of the grapes. Thus, fruit juices have a reduced nutritional profile compared to whole fruits.

Increases calorie/energy intake

Drinking your fruits tends to favor more energy consumption than eating your fruits. This is because it takes many more fruits to make a single juice serving. For instance, it takes about three medium-sized whole apples to make a cup of apple juice. While it may be more difficult to eat three apples in one sitting, drinking a cup of apple juice that contains the same three apples is way easier. Besides, people may also be tempted to drink more than one serving of juice, resulting in even more calories taken in at once. So, drinking two cups of apple juice in one sitting is equivalent to eating about six medium-sized apples, the latter being more unlikely than the former. Furthermore, removing fiber-rich peels and pulp in the juice-making process significantly decreases the soluble fiber's satiety effect, which helps reduce/control calorie consumption.

Increased intake of added sugars

Sugar consumption significantly increases with commercially prepared fruit juices. If you look at the nutrition profile of fruit juices that are not 100% fruit juice, you will see an item called "added sugars." This is sugar that is naturally not present in the fruit, or fruits used to make the juice. Sugars are added to make the juices taste sweet and this is why you would probably have noticed that freshly squeezed orange juice does not taste as sweet as commercially produced orange juice drink or nectar. The picture below shows the nutrition profile of a 100% fruit juice (which has no added sugar) and a 15% fruit juice (which contains added sugar).

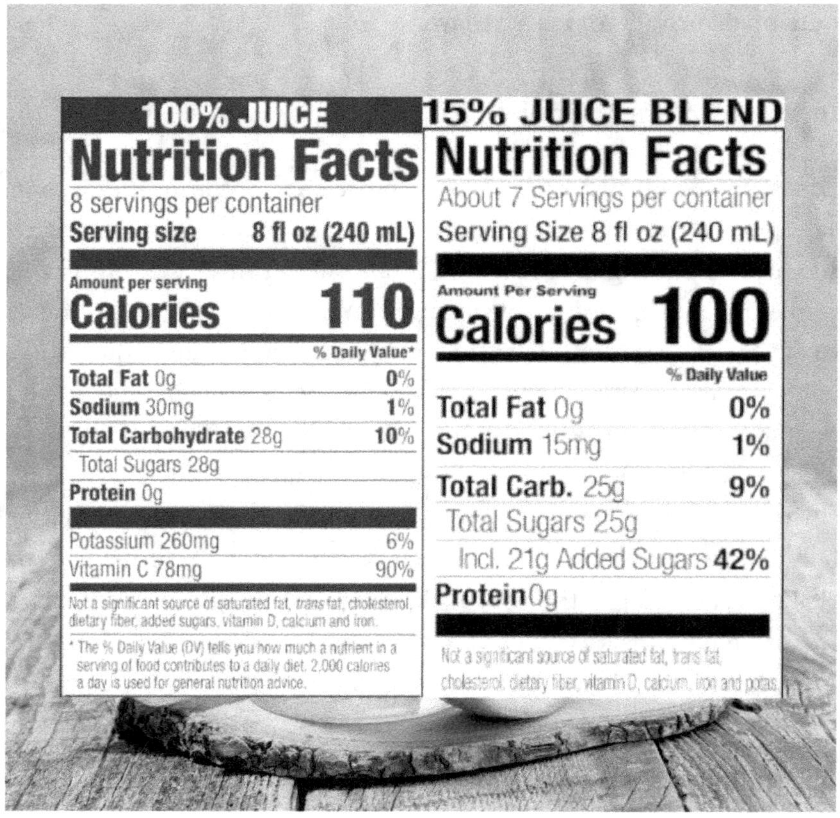

Fruit juice nutrition labels

Added sugars in sugar-sweetened beverages (including fruit drinks) is the main route to increased sugar intake in the diet. The increased prevalence of diabetes, which is currently the 8th leading cause of death in the United States is associated with increased intake of sugars through the diet. Research studies have proven a strong positive correlation between sugar-sweetened beverages and diabetes. Hence, consuming a lot of fruit drinks is an easy way to increase your risk of developing chronic diseases like diabetes.

Dental concerns

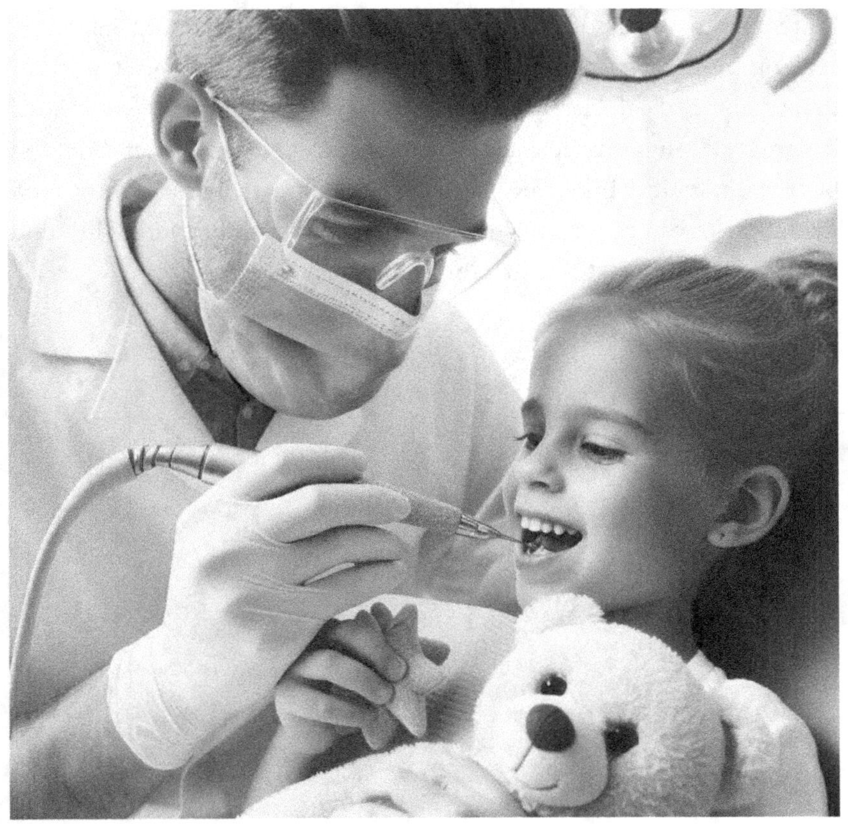

A little girl at a dental appointment

Like any other sugar-sweetened beverages, consuming plenty of fruit drinks can cause dental problems like dental carries and tooth decay, especially in children and teens under 18 years. Dental caries is the most common chronic disease children suffer in the United States, and sugar-sweetened beverages are a chief contributor to this problem. The National Health and Nutrition Education Survey (NHANES) data reports that sugar-sweetened beverages were the most common source of added sugars in the diet for children 2 – 18 years old in the United States. Two-thirds of children of this age group drink at least one serving of sugar-sweetened beverage every day, and about 7.3% of their daily total calories were reported to come from sugar-sweetened beverages. Sugar-sweetened beverages are defined as carbonated beverages, fruit drinks, energy drinks, and sports drinks. Untreated dental caries can cause pain and infections that can interfere with food intake and health status in the long run in severe cases.

4

Mid-Book Review Request Page

Title: **Make a Difference with Your Review**
Subtitle: **Unlock the Power of Consuming Fruits Right**

"When we guide others towards healthier food choices, we're not only feeding their bodies—we're fueling their potential." – Unknown

Helping others is one of the most amazing things we can do to foster our health and happiness. And you have a chance to do just that.

Imagine someone just like you – constantly trying to figure out whether eating fruits whole is better than drinking fruit juices. My mission is to make *Eating Vs Drinking Your Fruits* simple and accessible to everyone. But I cannot do it alone.

Most readers pick books based on reviews. So, please lend a hand to someone out there who wants to lead a healthy lifestyle by leaving a review.

Your review costs nothing and takes less than 60 seconds, yet it could change someone's fruit consumption pattern for life. Your words could help …

…one more person understand why eating whole fruits is better.

...one more person find a path to a healthier, happier life.

...one more parent make healthier fruit choices for their kids.

...one more family create nutritious habits that can last a lifetime.

Simply scan the QR code below to leave your review:

Thank you from the bottom of my heart! Now, let's get back to learning and growing together.

Your biggest fan, Margaret Tebo

5

Tips to Boost Fruit Consumption

Now that you have been enlightened on the potential health benefits of consuming fruits and that eating fruits whole has more health benefits than drinking fruit juices, the next matter of concern is optimizing your whole fruit consumption. As nutritious as fruits are, many find it hard to consume fruits regularly as they should. So, there must be an intentional effort on your part to make sure you are consuming your recommended fruit servings daily. Here are some helpful strategies.

Increase fruit visibility

If fruits are seen, they are much more likely to be eaten than if they are out of sight. Keeping fruits where you can easily see them makes grab-and-go an effortless process. Here are some tips to increase visibility.

1. Keep a fruit basket at the center of the kitchen or dining table. This makes fruits visible, accessible, and more likely to be eaten.
2. Place fruits on the front shelves of the fridge to make them visible and accessible. If they remain hidden at the back of the fridge they

might remain uneaten and end up rotten.

Incorporating whole fruits into the diet

Fruits can be eaten together with meals at different times of the day. Here are some ways to boost your fruit consumption during each meal.

Breakfast

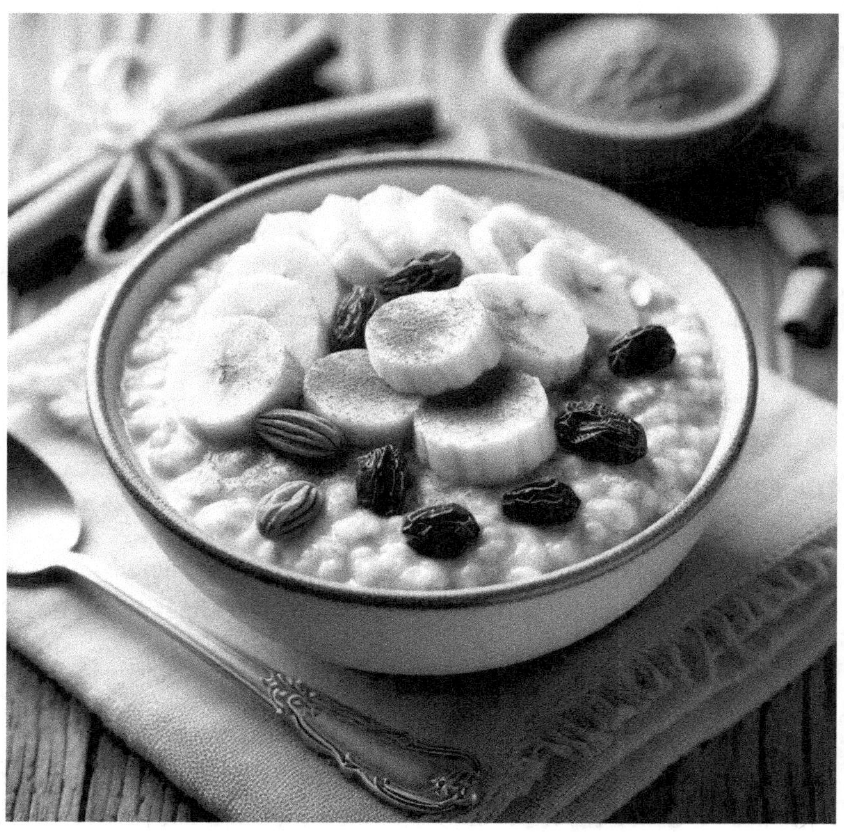

A bowl of oatmeal with raisins and slices of banana

1. Add fruits like bananas, cranberries, or raisins to your whole-grain cereals.
2. Slice apples, bananas, peaches, or pears and add them to your bowl of oatmeal.
3. Add berries or sliced pineapples, strawberries, or cherries to your yogurt (plain fat-free, or low-fat yogurt).
4. Add chopped apples or bananas to pancakes.
5. Eat fruits whole if you cannot add them directly to what you are having for breakfast.

Lunch

1. Choose a fruit salad for your entrée.
2. Add fruits like avocado to your sandwich.
3. Have some chopped whole fruits with your lunch.

Snack

1. Eat whole fruits for snacks. Keep fruits like apples, bananas, cherries, grapes, mandarins, and oranges easily available as grab-and-go fruits when you are on the run.
2. Chop different fruits and make a fruit salad bowl.
3. Add dried fruits like dates, raisins, apricots, and/or cranberries to nuts like almonds, pecans, and walnuts.
4. Chop fruits like bananas, grapes, and melon chunks to make fruit kabobs. Add an appropriate topping like yogurt or yogurt sauce. Alternatively, stack up red or green grapes and diced cheddar or mozzarella cheese for a great-tasting fruit kabobs.

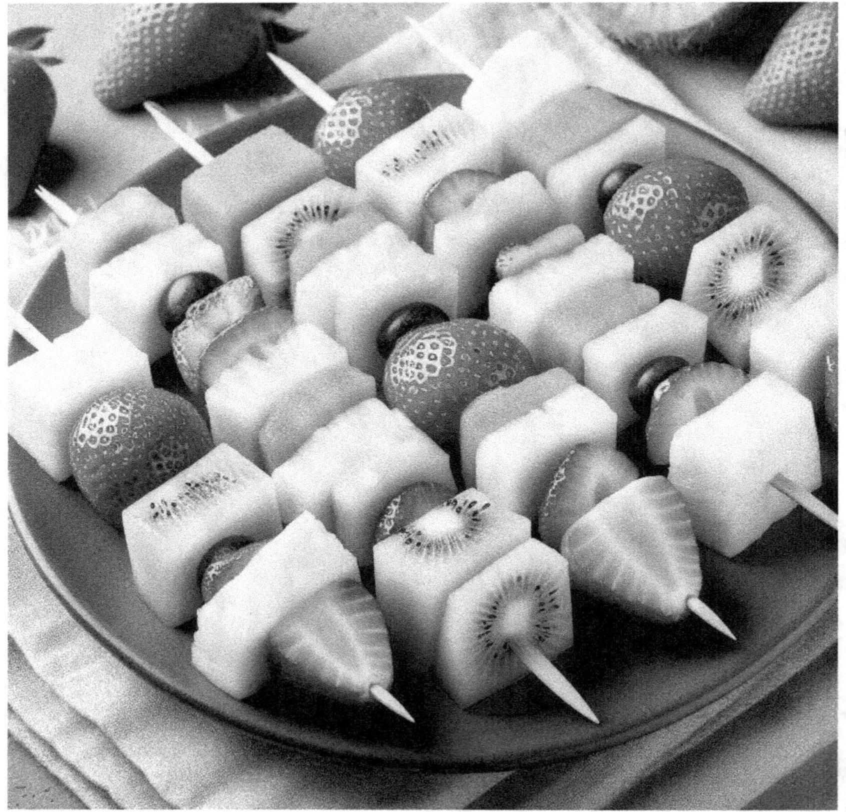

Fruit kabobs

Dinner

1. Have fruits fill a quarter of your plate.
2. Make a fruit salsa by chopping up a mixture of kiwis, peaches, strawberries, and apples. Then use the fruit salsa to top up chicken or fish recipes like salmon rice, or fish tacos.
3. Add to tossed salad fruits like apple wedges, grapes, grapefruit, dried cranberries or raisins.

4. Add fruits like blueberries to your burgers, avocado to your sandwiches, and strawberries to your quesadilla.
5. Add fruits like pineapple, dried cranberries, and apples to coleslaw.

6

Recommendations

To maximize the potential health benefits of consuming fruits, there are some recommendations from the MyPlate food model and the American Association of Diabetes.

General Recommendations on Fruit Consumption

1. Half your plate should be fruits and vegetables for optimal health benefits. This implies that a quarter of your plate should be fruits.
2. Consume at least half your recommended fruit servings as whole fruits rather than 100% fruit juice.
3. When consuming dried fruits, note that a cup contains many more calories than a cup of cut fresh whole fruits: one cup of fresh fruit is equivalent to half a cup of dried fruit.
4. When you shop for dried fruits, go more for unsweetened dried fruits rather than their sweetened counterparts, otherwise, your dried fruits will become another route for increased sugar intake just like sweetened fruit juices. So, always look out for the "added sugar" item on the nutrition profile of the fruit packet. A pack of sweetened dried cranberries can have over 50% of its total sugar

as added sugars.

5. If you consume canned fruits, choose the unsweetened and less sodium options. The goal is to minimize the consumption of added sugars and salt.

6. Get a personalized fruit consumption plan by visiting the MyPlate website at https://www.myplate.gov/myplate-plan. You will be asked to enter your age, sex, height, weight, and physical activity level, to get your customized plan.

Recommendations for Fruit Juice Consumption

Here are some recommendations to guide you to get the most out of drinking your fruits.

1. Drink 100% fruit juice. The MyPlate food model includes 100% fruit juice as part of the fruit group, so if you desire to drink your fruits it is better to aim more for 100% fruit juice. You can treat yourself or your kids to fruit drinks occasionally, but it is not advisable health-wise to consistently drink plenty of fruit drinks because of added sugars and low crude fruit content.

2. Moderate your fruit juice consumption. The MyPlate food model recommends that people over 14 years consume at most one cup of 100% fruit juice a day. As discussed earlier, drinking your fruit makes it easy to overconsume calories and natural sugars, so keeping your consumption to no more than one cup is a great way to keep your consumption in check.

3. Make smoothies. Instead of juicing all the time, try making a smoothie now and then. Smoothies are a healthier way of drinking your fruits than juices since they are just blends of whole fruits. With smoothies, you consume fiber-rich peels and pulp, and many cocktail options are also available. Besides, smoothies are very

filling because they contain fiber, and the satiety effect of fiber also kicks in when you drink a smoothie.

7

Conclusion

The fruit group is an integral part of any healthy diet plan. Fruits are a good source of minerals and vitamins that the body needs daily for optimal growth, development, function, and repair. Fruits are also rich in fiber, which plays a crucial role in maintaining our microbiota balance, further fostering digestive health and enhancing overall body immunity. Additionally, fiber helps with weight loss/management, blood sugar control, and blood cholesterol reduction. Furthermore, fruits contain compounds like carotenoids and polyphenols which exhibit strong antioxidant and anti-inflammatory activities that protect the body cells from oxidative damage. As such they help to reduce the risk of development of certain cancers and chronic diseases like arthritis, diabetes, and heart disease.

The most popular ways people consume fruits include eating them whole or drinking them in commercially manufactured or homemade fruit juices. Eating your fruits whole bestows more health benefits than drinking your fruits. Whole fruits have more dietary fiber, antioxidants, polyphenols, minerals, and vitamins. Fruit juices tend to contain less of these nutrients because of the removal of peels and pulp during the fruit juice manufacturing process. Besides, drinking your fruits tends to favor more calories and sugar intake, leading to a rapid rise in blood sugar levels and weight gain in the long run. Fruit drinks are typically packed with sugar and have the least nutrients due to their low crude juice content. The regular consumption of fruit drinks increases the risk of developing chronic diseases like dental caries in children and teens, and obesity and diabetes in both children and adults.

The MyPlate food model recommends that people eat more of their fruits whole than drink them as fruit juice. The fruit juice recommended as part of a healthy plate is 100% fruit juice and drinking should be moderated to at most one cup a day because of higher natural sugar content.

So, depending on where you are in your health and lifestyle journey, adopting the best practices can enable you to maximize the amazing health benefits of fruit consumption. Creating a good balance between eating whole fruits and consuming some fruit juice as MyPlate recommends, should enable you to enjoy the best of both worlds.

8

End of Book Review Page

Title: **Make a Difference with Your Review**
Subtitle: **Unlock the Power of Consuming Fruits Right**

Now that you have everything you need to make the best choices between eating whole fruits and drinking fruit juices, it's time to pass on your newfound knowledge and help others discover the same benefits you just did.

The simple act of leaving your honest opinion of this book on Amazon will show other health-conscious readers where they can find the information they're looking for and inspire them to make healthier food choices as well.

Simply scan the QR code below to leave your review:

Thank you very much for your help. The journey to healthy eating is kept alive when we pass on the knowledge we have received—and you're helping me do just that.

9

References

References

1. (N.d.). Lipid.Org. Retrieved July 12, 2024, from https://www.lipid.org/sites/default/files/adding_soluble_fiber_final_0.pdf

2. 11 Foods that Lower Cholesterol - Harvard Health Publishing. (2024, March 26). Harvard Health. https://www.health.harvard.edu/heart-health/11-foods-that-lower-cholesterol

3. Bhosale, P. B., Ha, S. E., Vetrivel, P., Kim, H. H., Kim, S. M., & Kim, G. S. (2020). Functions of polyphenols and its anticancer properties in biomedical research: a narrative review. Translational Cancer Research, 9(12), 7619. https://doi.org/10.21037/tcr-20-2359

4. Bromelain. (n.d.). NCCIH. Retrieved July 6, 2024, from https://www.nccih.nih.gov/health/bromelain

5. Brouns, F., Theuwissen, E., Adam, A., Bell, M., Berger, A., & Mensink, R. P. (2012). Cholesterol-lowering properties of different pectin types in mildly hyper-cholesterolemic men and women. European Journal of Clinical Nutrition, 66(5), 591–599. https://doi.org/10.1038/ejcn.2011.208

6. Calderón-Oliver, M., & Ponce-Alquicira, E. (2018). Fruits: A source of polyphenols and health benefits. In A. M. Grumezescu & A. M. Holban (Eds.), Natural and Artificial Flavoring Agents and Food Dyes (pp. 189–228). Elsevier.

7. CDC. (2024, May 22). Fiber: The Carb That Helps You Manage. Diabetes. https://www.cdc.gov/diabetes/healthy-eating/fiber-hel ps-diabetes.html

8. Chi, D. L., & Scott, J. M. (2019). Added sugar and dental caries in children: A scientific update and future steps. Dental Clinics of North America, 63(1), 17–33. https://doi.org/10.1016/j.cden.201 8.08.003

9. Eating, Diet, & Nutrition for Constipation. (2022, July 20). National Institute of Diabetes and Digestive and Kidney Diseases; NIDDK - National Institute of Diabetes and Digestive and Kidney Diseases. https://www.niddk.nih.gov/health-information/digesti ve-diseases/constipation/eating-diet-nutrition

10. Focus on Whole Fruits. (n.d.). Myplate.Gov. Retrieved July 9, 2024, from https://www.myplate.gov/tip-sheet/focus-whole-fruits

11. FoodData Central. (n.d.). Usda.Gov. Retrieved July 3, 2024, from https://fdc.nal.usda.gov/fdc-app.html#/food-details/325430/nut rients

12. FoodData Central. (n.d.). Usda.Gov. Retrieved July 3, 2024, from https://fdc.nal.usda.gov/fdc-app.html#/food-details/173946/nut rients

13. Hollis, J. H. (2018). The effect of mastication on food intake, satiety and body weight. Physiology & Behavior, 193(Pt B), 242–245. https://doi.org/10.1016/j.physbeh.2018.04.027

14. How to Eat More Fruit and Vegetables. (n.d.). Www.Heart.Org. Retrieved July 9, 2024, from https://www.heart.org/en/healthy-li ving/healthy-eating/add-color/how-to-eat-more-fruits-and-vege tables

15. Hussain, T., Kalhoro, D. H., & Yin, Y. (2022). Identification of nutritional composition and antioxidant activities of fruit peels as a potential source of nutraceuticals. Frontiers in Nutrition, 9, 1065698. https://doi.org/10.3389/fnut.2022.1065698

16. Hydrating for Health. (n.d.). NIH News in Health. Retrieved July 3, 2024, from https://newsinhealth.nih.gov/2023/05/hydrating-health

17. Is fruit juice healthier than whole fruit? (n.d.). Science Questions with Surprising Answers. Retrieved July 7, 2024, from https://wtamu.edu/~cbaird/sq/2013/12/02/is-fruit-juice-healthier-than-whole-fruit/

18. Kenneth R, F. (2024). Table 10. [Fiber Content of Selected Fruits]. MDText.com, Inc.

19. Ko, J.-H., Sethi, G., Um, J.-Y., Shanmugam, M. K., Arfuso, F., Kumar, A. P., Bishayee, A., & Ahn, K. S. (2017). The Role of Resveratrol in Cancer Therapy. International Journal of Molecular Sciences, 18(12). https://doi.org/10.3390/ijms18122589

20. Kumar, A., P N., Kumar, M., Jose, A., Tomer, V., Oz, E., Proestos, C., Zeng, M., Elobeid, T., K, S., & Oz, F. (2023). Major phytochemicals: Recent advances in health benefits and extraction method. Molecules (Basel, Switzerland), 28(2). https://doi.org/10.3390/molecules28020887

21. Machado, C. L. R., Crespo-Lopez, M. E., Augusto-Oliveira, M., Arrifano, G. de P., Macchi, B. de M., Lopes-Araújo, A., Santos-Sacramento, L., Souza-Monteiro, J. R., Alvarez-Leite, J. I., & Souza, C. B. A. de. (2021). Eating in the Amazon: Nutritional status of the riverine populations and possible nudge interventions. Foods (Basel, Switzerland), 10(5), 1015. https://doi.org/10.3390/foods10051015

22. News briefs: Eating fruit is better for you than drinking fruit juice. (2013, December 1). Harvard Health. https://www.health.harvard.

edu/staying-healthy/news-briefs-eating-fruit-is-better-for-you-t
han-drinking-fruit-juice

23. Over time, racial and ethnic gaps in dietary fiber consumption per 1,000 calories have widened. (n.d.). Usda.Gov. Retrieved July 7, 2024, from http://www.ers.usda.gov/data-products/chart-gallery /gallery/chart-detail/?chartId=106189

24. Polyphenols: food sources and bioavailability. (n.d.). Oup.Com. Retrieved July 2, 2024, from https://academic.oup.com/view-larg e/109820549?login=false

25. Potassium and hypertension - UpToDate. (n.d.). Uptodate.Com. Retrieved July 2, 2024, from https://www.uptodate.com/contents /potassium-and-hypertension

26. Principles and practices of small - and medium - scale fruit juice processing. (n.d.). Fao.Org. Retrieved July 12, 2024, from https://w ww.fao.org/4/Y2515E/y2515e03.htm

27. Rebello, C. J., O'Neil, C. E., & Greenway, F. L. (2016). Dietary fiber and satiety: the effects of oats on satiety. Nutrition Reviews, 74(2), 131–147. https://doi.org/10.1093/nutrit/nuv063

28. USDA MyPlate Fruit Group – One of the Five Food Groups. (n.d.). Myplate.Gov. Retrieved June 26, 2024, from https://www.myplat e.gov/eat-healthy/fruits

29. Valder, S., & Brinkmann, C. (2022). Is intake of fruit juice useful in exercise-induced hypoglycemia prevention in individuals with type 1 diabetes mellitus? Frontiers in Endocrinology, 13, 1045639. https://doi.org/10.3389/fendo.2022.1045639

30. Vitamin C. (n.d.). Nih.Gov. Retrieved July 2, 2024, from https://o ds.od.nih.gov/factsheets/VitaminC-Consumer/

31. Wang, D. D., Li, Y., Bhupathiraju, S. N., Rosner, B. A., Sun, Q., Giovannucci, E. L., Rimm, E. B., Manson, J. E., Willett, W. C., Stampfer, M. J., & Hu, F. B. (2021). Fruit and vegetable intake and mortality: Results from 2 prospective cohort studies of US men

and women and a meta-analysis of 26 cohort studies. Circulation, 143(17), 1642–1654. https://doi.org/10.1161/circulationaha.120. 048996

32. What Can Hunter-Gatherers Teach Us about Staying Healthy? (2019, April 21). Duke Global Health Institute. https://globalhealt h.duke.edu/news/what-can-hunter-gatherers-teach-us-about-sta ying-healthy

33. Zhang, Y.-J., Li, S., Gan, R.-Y., Zhou, T., Xu, D.-P., & Li, H.-B. (2015). Impacts of Gut Bacteria on Human Health and Diseases. International Journal of Molecular Sciences, 16(4), 7493. https://d oi.org/10.3390/ijms16047493

10

Medical Disclaimer

lthough this book presents research findings and medical insights, the content of this book is solely for information and education purposes. It should by no means replace professional and medical advice or consultations with health care professionals.

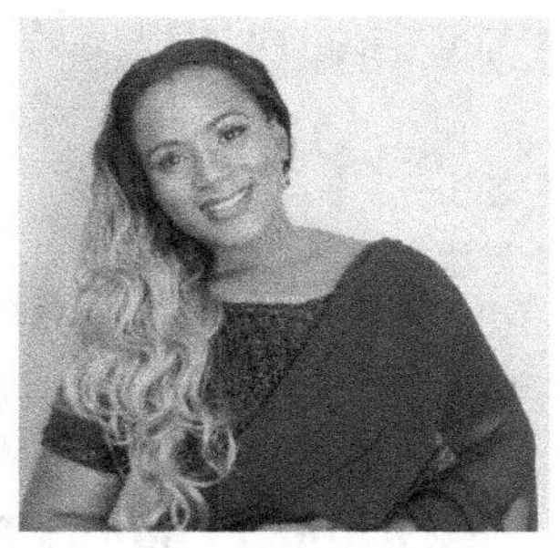

About the Author

Margaret Bechem Epse Tebo is a Nutritionist who holds a Master of Science degree in Nutrition. She has co-authored a few academic journals and is currently a freelance researcher and writer in Nutrition, Health, and Wellness on Fiverr. Over her three-plus years on Fiverr, she has written hundreds of articles for food and dietary supplement companies, as well as nutrition and health blogs. Additionally, she runs a food and nutrition blog called NUTRIAWE (https://nutriawe.com/) where she writes on health and wellness. She also deep dives into the awesomeness of good nutrition by proposing delicious healthy recipes.

You can connect with me on:
🌐 https://nutriawe.com

Also by Margaret Tebo

As a nutritionist, I focus on content that provides nutrition information to enhance knowledge and help people make healthier food choices.

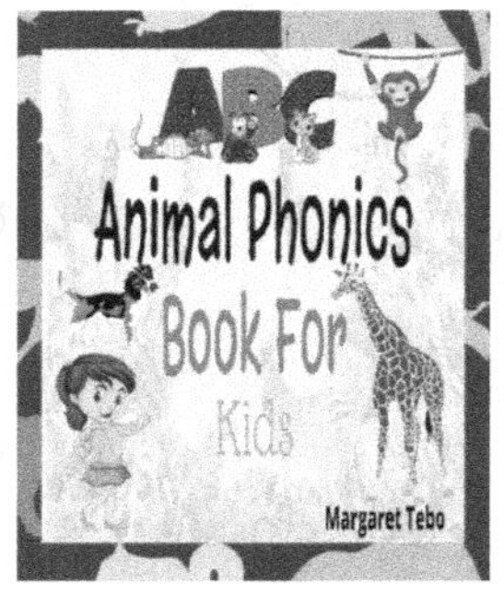

ABC Animal Phonics Books For Kids

This book is the perfect tool to teach your kids the alphabet as it contains the different animals of the world from A to Z. In addition, it has the English language pronunciation for each animal to enhance learning and a fun fact about each animal, particularly their feeding habit.

ABC FRUITS & VEGETABLES PHONICS BOOK FOR KIDS

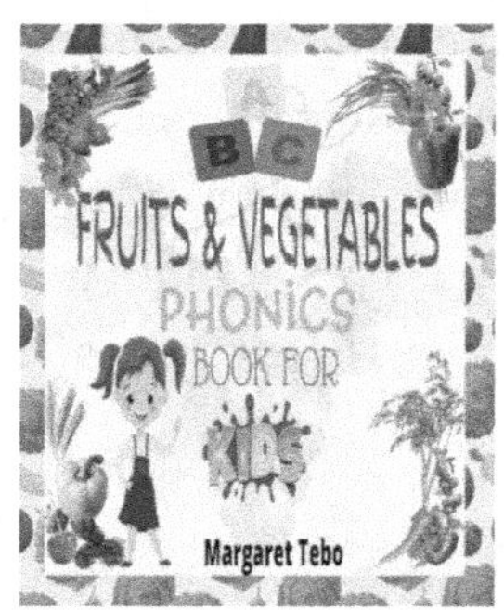

This book is a great learning tool for kids as it contains everyday fruits and vegetables from A to Z, to optimize learning. It also has a nutrition education element as calorie information for all the fruits and vegetables used is provided per 100-gram serving.

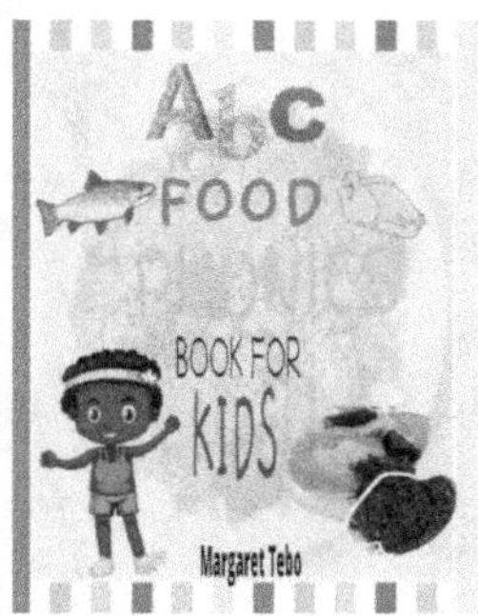

Abc FOOD PHONICS BOOK FOR KIDS

This book is more than just an alphabet-learning book for kids. It contains the A to Z of the Cameroon cuisine, with explanations of what each meal is made of, the scientific names of the major ingredients used, and the health benefits of key nutrients present in these major ingredients. This book is a great cultural learning tool for young kids, older kids, and parents as well.